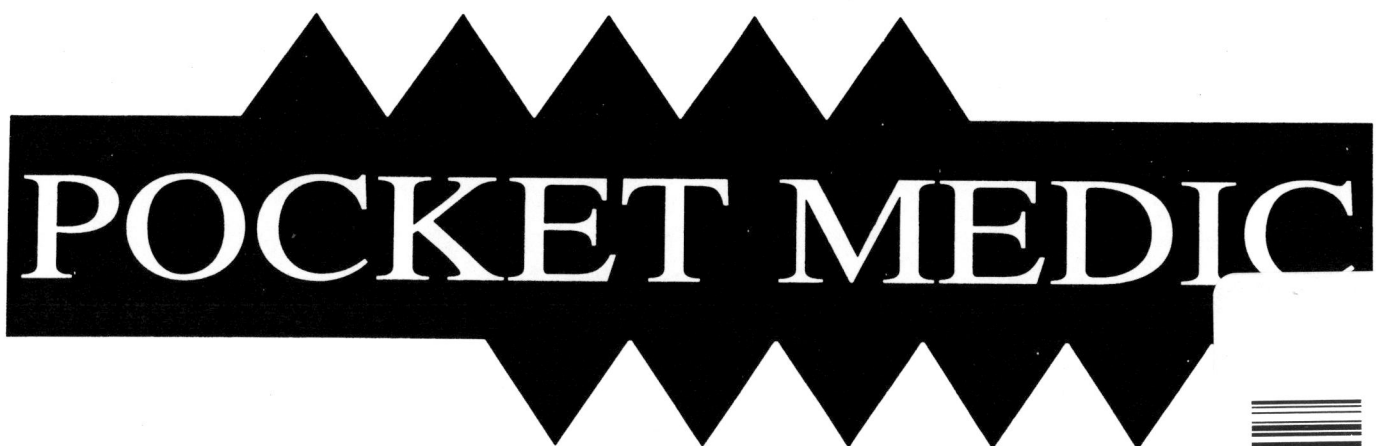

POCKET MEDIC

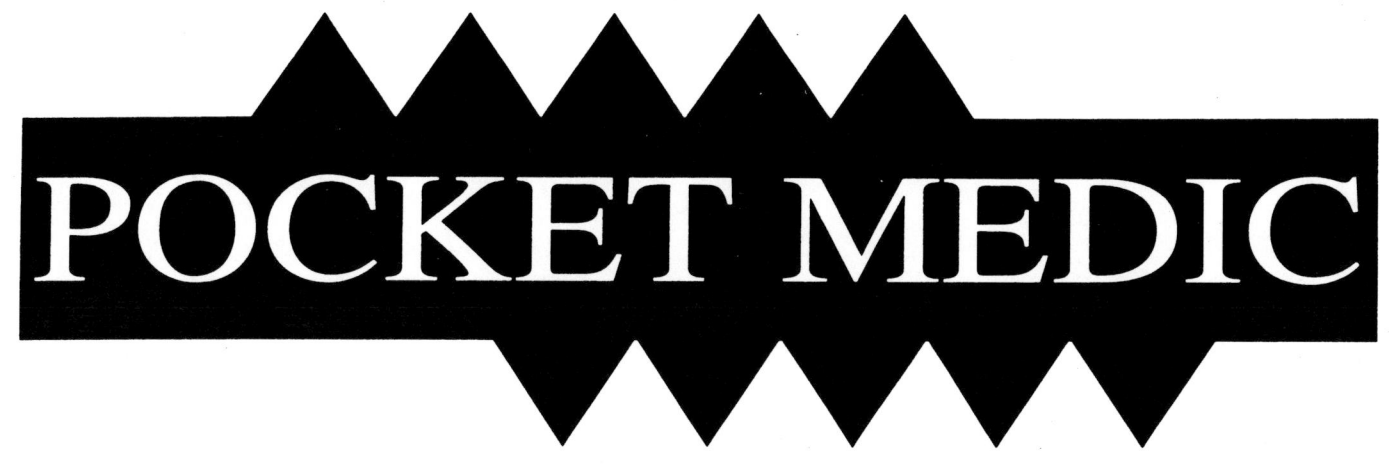

POCKET MEDIC

THE INDISPENSABLE FIRST AID GUIDE

PALADIN PRESS
BOULDER, COLORADO

Pocket Medic:
The Indispensable First Aid Guide

Copyright © 1992 by Paladin Press

ISBN 10: 0-87364-662-2
ISBN 13: 978-0-87364-662-8
Printed in the United States of America

Published by Paladin Press, a division of
Paladin Enterprises, Inc.
Gunbarrel Tech Center
7077 Winchester Circle
Boulder, Colorado 80301 USA
+1.303.443.7250

Direct inquiries and/or orders to the above address.

Visit our Web site at www.paladin-press.com

TABLE OF CONTENTS

Part 1--LIFESAVING MEASURES

Part 2--SPECIAL FIRST AID MEASURES

Part 3--FIRST AID FOR COMMON EMERGENCIES

Aid in Time - - - - - - - - -

Since a medic cannot be with every soldier, your life and the lives of other soldiers may depend upon how much you know about first aid.

First aid is the emergency or lifesaving care given to a sick, injured, or wounded person when a medically trained person is not immediately available. Without this emergency care, a sick, injured, or wounded person may not live until he can receive medical treatment. It is important that everyone know how to apply lifesaving first aid measures, especially the soldier on the training field or battlefield.

This pocket manual is designed to be a handy guide when an emergency arises. For this reason, it contains only essential information about real emergencies which you may face and should be able to handle. To learn how to apply all first aid measures, you should read FM 21-11.

PART I

Lifesaving Measures:

A   **Open airway and restore breathing and heartbeat**   Lack of oxygen intake (through breathing and heartbeat) leads to death in very few minutes.

B   **Stop bleeding**   Life cannot continue without adequate volume of blood to carry oxygen to tissues.

C   **Prevent shock**   Unless shock is prevented or corrected, death may result even though injury would not otherwise be fatal.

D   **Dress and bandage wounds to avoid infection**   Healing of wound and recovery depend to great extent upon how well wound was protected from contamination initially.

BASIC GUIDES

1. Examine promptly and calmly for:

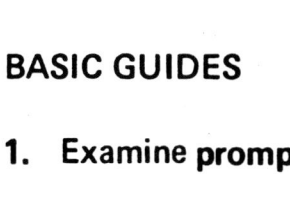

Absence of breathing — See no movement of chest — OR — Feel no air from nose or mouth — OR — Hear no air from nose or mouth

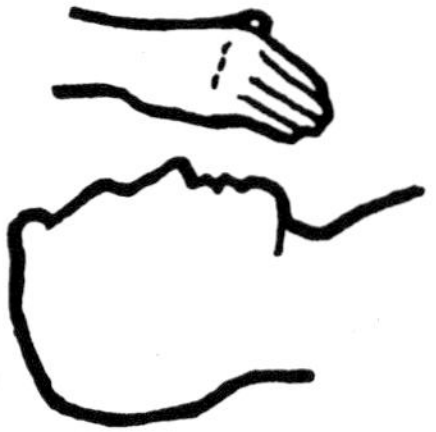

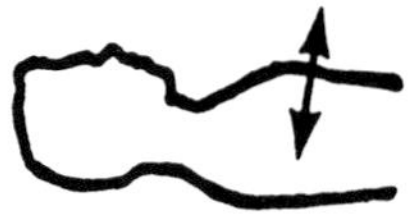

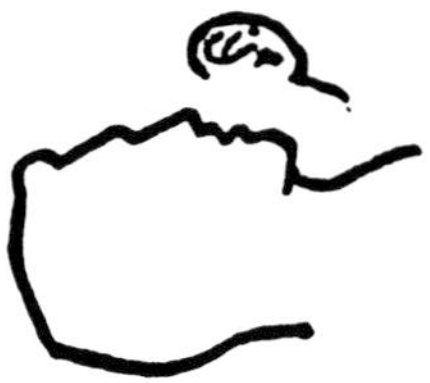

Absence of heartbeat 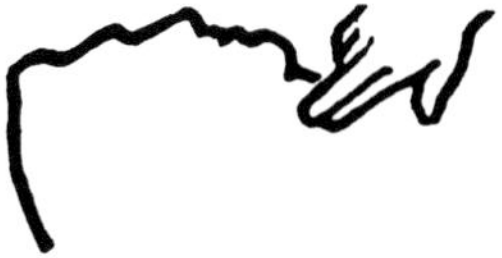 — Feel no pulse with tips of fingers (not thumb) on neck at side of windpipe

Presence of bleeding — See blood. Spurting blood means bleeding from artery (not vein or capillary).

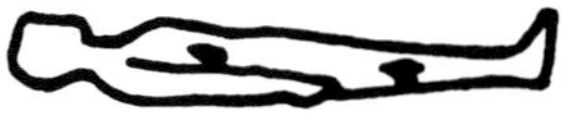

2. Apply lifesaving measures A and B instantly.

If no sign of breathing . . . . Open airway (A).

If still no sign of breathing . . . . Start artificial respiration (A).*

If no pulse or only very weak, irregular pulse . . . . . Start closed-chest heart massage with artificial respiration (A).*

If bleeding . . . . Apply pressure (B).

3. Re-examine immediately head-to-toe and front-to-back for:

Other injuries- - - Fractures, injuries without associated wounds, etc.

Signs of shock - - -Early signs: Restlessness, thirst, pale skin, rapid heartbeat. May be excited or appear calm and very tired; may be sweating although skin is cool and clammy.
Signs when shock becomes worse: Fast breaths or gasps; staring into space; blotchy or bluish skin, especially around mouth.

4. Apply lifesaving measures C and D promptly.

Apply shock prevention and control measures (C).
Dress and bandage wounds to avoid infection (D).

5. Arrange evacuation to nearest medical treatment facility.

*Continue until the person regains consciousness, until you are relieved by medically trained person, or for at least 45 minutes in the absence of all life signs.

(To act incorrectly can be just as serious or fatal to a wounded soldier as the failure to administer a lifesaving measure.)

1.   Do not let soldier remain on his back if he is unconscious or has face or neck wound.

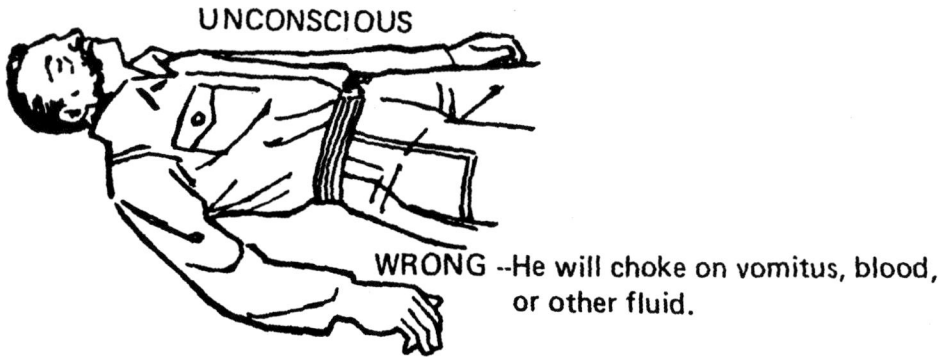

UNCONSCIOUS

WRONG --He will choke on vomitus, blood, or other fluid.

2.   Do not pull or tear clothing from injured soldier.

3.   Do not touch or try to clean dirty wounds, including burns.

4.   Do not remove dressings and bandages once they have been placed over wound.

5.   Do not loosen tourniquet once it has been applied.

6. Do not move soldier with fracture until it has been properly splinted unless necessary to save his life.

7. Do not give fluids to soldier who is unconscious, nauseated, or vomiting or has abdominal or neck wound.

8. Do not permit head to be lower than body when soldier has head injury.

9. Do not try to push protruding intestines or brain tissue back into wound.

10. Do not put any medication on burns.

11. Do not try to give first aid measures which are unnecessary or beyond your capabilities.

12. Do not fail to resupply your first aid case with items used from it.

OPEN AIRWAY (A)

For air to flow to and from lungs, upper airway must be open.

Airway closed by tongue

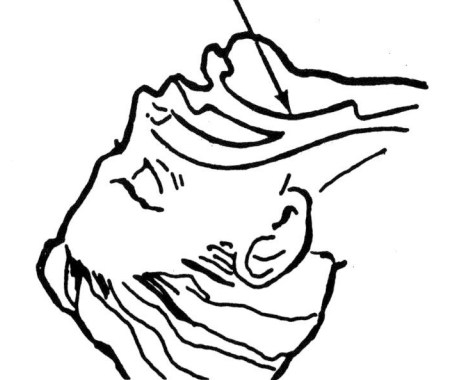

Airway opened by extending neck

To open airway, place soldier on his back with neck extended and head in chin-up position.

(If a rolled blanket, poncho, or similar object is readily available, place it under his shoulders to help maintain this position.)

To open airway farther, place your thumb in soldier's mouth, grasp his lower jaw, and lift it forward.

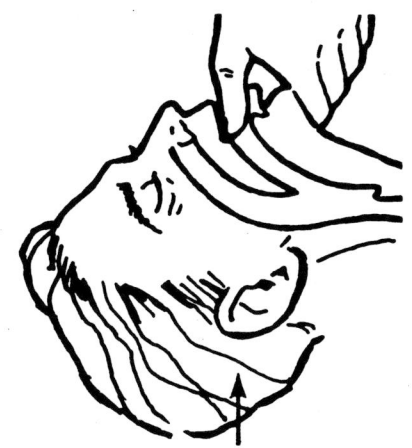

Airway opened farther by adjusting jaw

If you cannot get your thumb into his mouth, grasp angles of lower jaw with both hands and lift jaw forcibly forward; then open his lips by pushing lower lip toward chin with your thumbs.

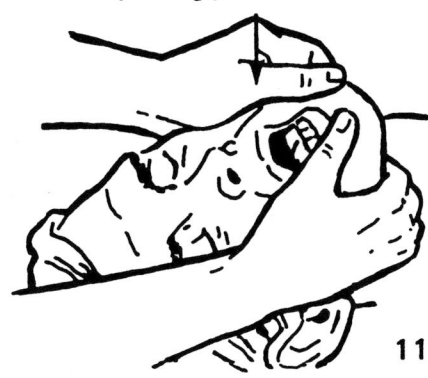

11

Mouth-to-Mouth Method of Artificial Respiration (A)

(This method is used except when soldier has a crushed face or is in toxic environment.)

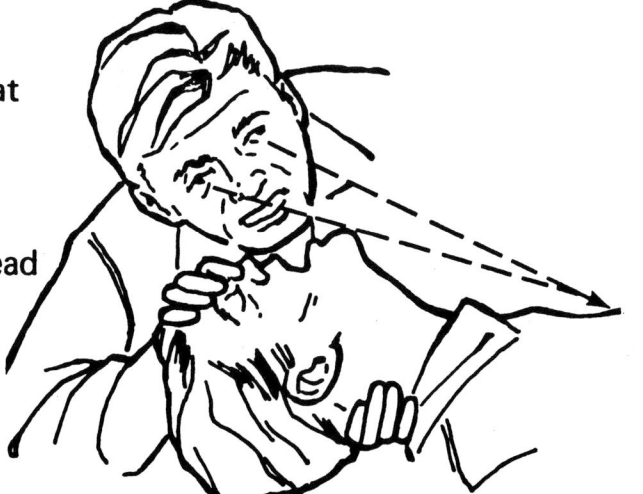

1. With soldier lying on back, position yourself at side of his head.

2. Place one hand behind his neck to keep his head in a face-up, tilted-back position. Pinch his nostrils with thumb and index finger of other hand and let same hand press on his forehead to keep head tilted backward.

For adults: First 4 breaths —Full and quick
Thereafter ------   1 every 5 seconds
For children: Puffs of air from cheeks

3. Take deep breath and place mouth (in airtight seal) around soldier's mouth; then blow forcefully as you observe his chest.

   (If his chest does not rise, adjust his jaw and blow harder, making sure air is not leaking from his mouth or nose. If chest still does not rise, turn his head to one side, run your fingers down inside of lower cheeks, over base of tongue, and across back of throat to remove vomitus, mucus, or foreign bodies. If airway is still not clear, roll him onto his side; using heel of hand, deliver sharp blows between his shoulder blades to dislodge foreign body. An alternate method for dislodging foreign body is Heimlich maneuver B, page 52.)

4. When soldier's chest rises, remove your mouth from his mouth and listen for return of air from his lungs. If returning air is noisy, lift his jaw.

5. After each exhalation of air, pinch his nose again and blow another deep breath. First 4 breaths should be full and quick (except for children); thereafter, the rate is once every 5 seconds. Insure adequate ventilation on each breath by observing his chest rise and fall and by hearing and feeling air from his lungs.

6. As soldier starts to breathe, adjust timing to assist him. (If abdomen bulges, apply gentle pressure on abdomen with hand at frequent intervals between inflations.)

NOTE: The mouth-to-nose method is performed in the same way except you blow into his nose while you pinch his lips closed with one hand.

Chest-Pressure Arm-Lift Method of Artificial Respiration (A)

(For use when mouth-to-mouth method cannot be used because of a crushed face)

1. Clear soldier's airway and position him on his back with face up. Place rolled blanket or similar object under his shoulders so his head drops in chin-up position.

2. Kneel on one knee at his head and place other foot against his shoulder.
   (May alternate knee and foot positions to reduce discomfort.)

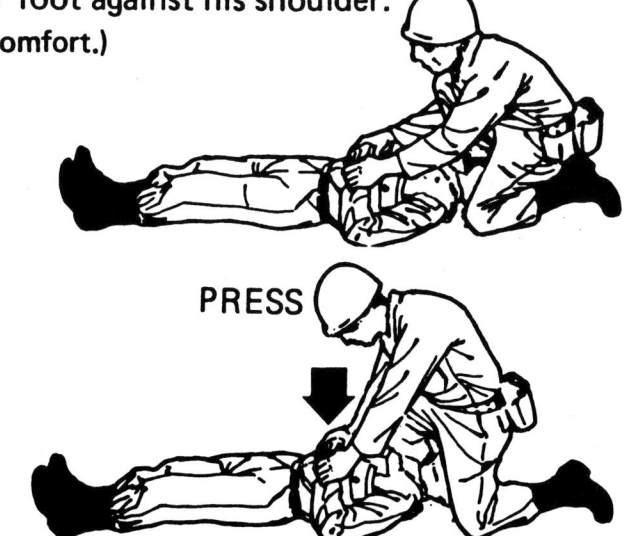

PRESS

3. Hold soldier's hands over his lower ribs, rock forward and exert steady, uniform pressure almost directly downward until meet firm resistance. This pressure forces air from his lungs.

4. Lift his arms vertically upward and stretch them backward as far as possible. This process of lifting and stretching his arms increases size of his chest and draws air into his lungs.

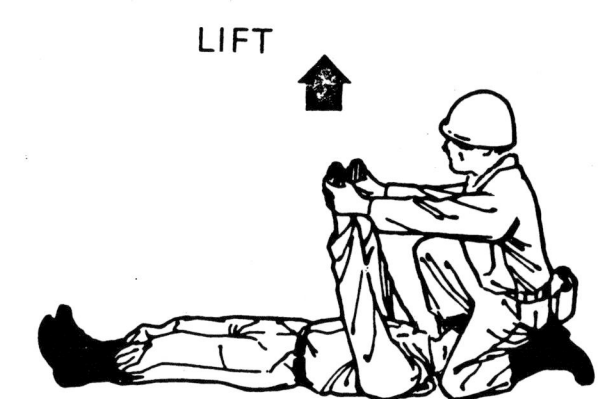

LIFT

5. Replace his hands on chest and repeat cycle: PRESS, LIFT, STRETCH, REPLACE.

Give 10 to 12 cycles per minute at a steady, uniform rate. Give count of equal lengths to PRESS, LIFT, and STRETCH steps. Perform REPLACE step as quickly as possible.

6. As he attempts to breathe, adjust timing to assist him.

STRETCH

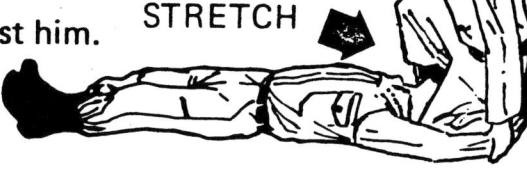

RESTORE HEARTBEAT (A)

Closed-chest Heart Massage With Artificial Respiration. (A)

(To keep blood flowing to brain and other vital organs until heart begins beating normally again.)

1. Prepare soldier for artificial respiration. (Breathing stops before or soon after heart stops.) Place him on solid surface. Elevate his legs about 6 inches by placing his pack or another suitable object under his feet.

2. Position yourself close to his side. Place heel of one hand on lower half of breastbone with fingers spread and raised. Place other hand on top of first hand. (Use only one hand for child and only fingers for infant.)

3. Bring shoulders directly over breatbone; keep arms straight; press breastbone down only 1½ to 2 inches. (More than 2 inches may fracture breastbone. If child or infant, press only lightly.)

4. Release pressure immediately, keeping hands in place. Continue with proper timing, using either two rescuers or one rescuer.

Two Rescuers

Compressions --- **1 per second** (60/minute)

Timing **for natural rhythm--** Count aloud: one 1000, two 1000, three 1000, four 1000, five 1000.

Compress as say, "one," "two," "three," "four," "five." Release as say, "one thousand."

Repeat count without pause for breath to be blown into airway.

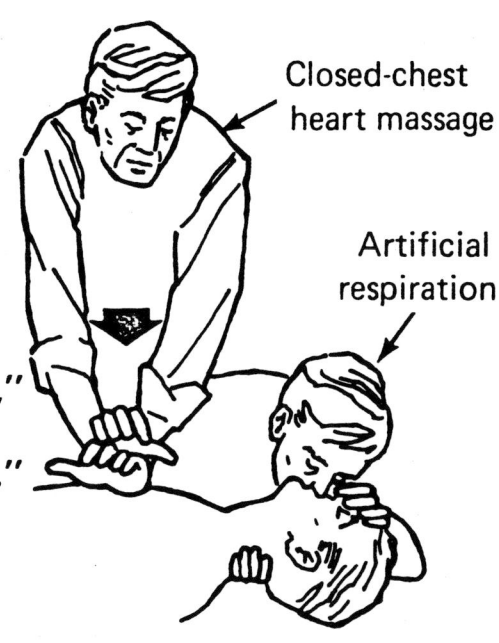

Closed-chest heart massage

Artificial respiration

Inflations -- **1 after each 5 compressions (5: 1 ratio)**

Timing: **At the 1000 following five, blow deep breath into airway.**

This timing is important, as any interruption in compression causes drop in blood flow and blood pressure to zero.

NOTE ILLUSTRATION: One rescuer should be on each side of the soldier—not both on the same side.

Closed-Chest Heart Massage With Artificial Respiration (con't) (A)

Two Rescuers -- Position Switch

When one rescuer becomes fatigued, he can switch positions with the other rescuer without any significant interruption in 5:1 rhythm:

Rescuer giving artificial respiration:

After inflate lungs, move to other side; place hands in air next to other rescuer's hands; and after two-1000 or three-1000 count, take over the compressions.

Rescuer giving closed-chest heart massage:

After other rescuer takes over compressions, move to other side and blow the next breath on the one-thousand following five.

Compressions - - - **80 per minute**

Inflations - - - - **2 (quick but full) after each 15 heart compressions (15: 2 ratio)**

Timing - - - **Count aloud: 1 and 2 and 3 and 4 and 5 and, 1 and 2 and 3 and 4 and 10 and, 1 and 2 and 3 and 4 and 15.**

Compress as say the numbers.
Release as say "and."
Blow after count of 15 two deep breaths into airway in rapid succession without allowing full return of air.

Repeat count as continue resuscitation.

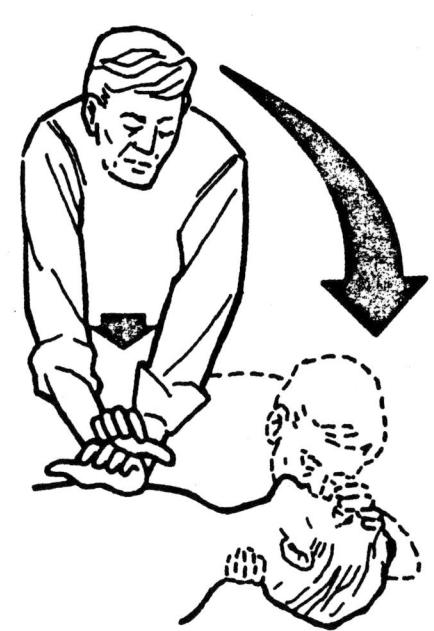

STOP BLEEDING (B)

Uncontrolled bleeding leads to shock and finally death.

Application of pressure dressings with hand pressure is preferred method to control bleeding.

Elevation of wounded limb and application of digital pressure are used in addition to pressure dressings, as appropriate.

Tourniquet is applied to control bleeding from limb only after all other methods have failed.

Use of tourniquet may be the only way you can stop bleeding from a major artery or from multiple arteries when limb has been crushed or amputated.

1. Check for more than one wound.

A missile usually makes smaller wound where it enters than where it exits.

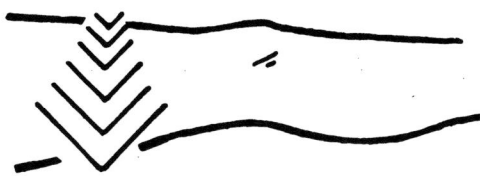

2. Cut and lift clothing from wound.

Tearing clothing results in rough handling of injured part.

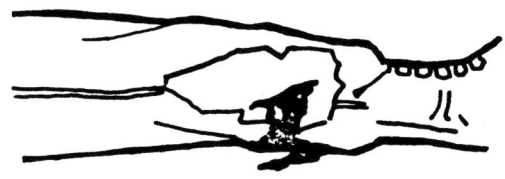

3. Prevent further contamination of wound. Don't touch wound.

Any attempt to clean wound only contaminates it more. If found dirty, leave dirty.

4. Cover wound and apply pressure. (page 22)

Pressure Dressings (B)
(Preferred method)

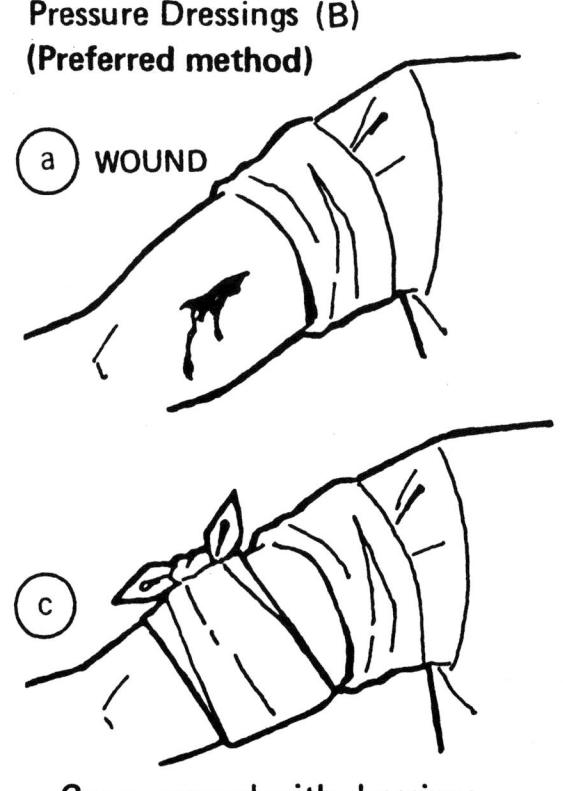

(a) WOUND

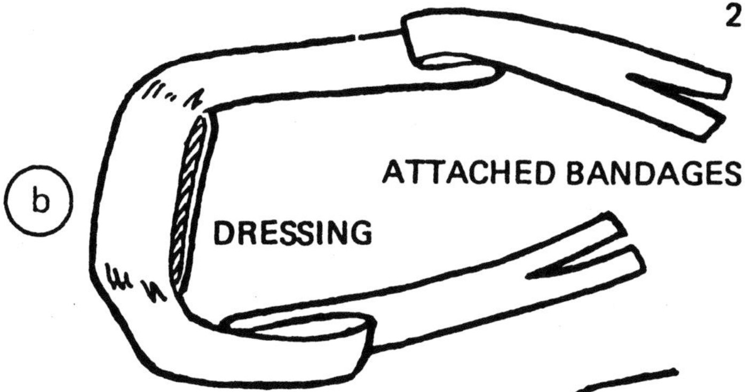

(b) DRESSING   ATTACHED BANDAGES

(c)
Cover wound with dressing; apply pressure with bandages.

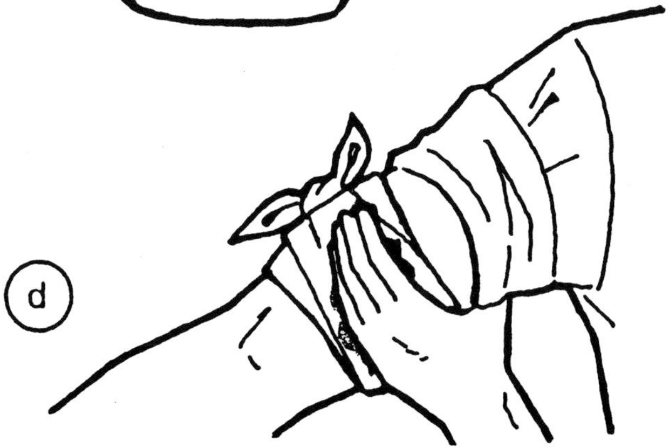

(d)
If bleeding continues, press wound with hand for 5-10 minutes.

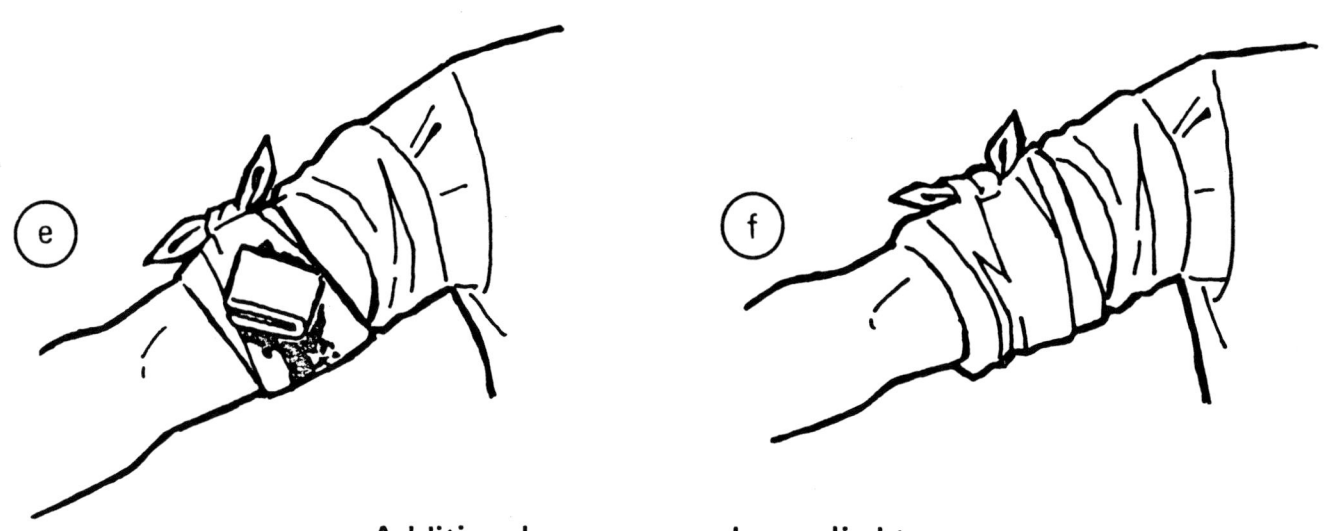

Additional pressure can be applied to wound with thick pad (rag) firmly secured with cravat or other strip of material.

NOTE: If no first aid dressing is available, use any available cloth. Once dressing is applied, don't remove.

Elevation of Wounded Limb (B)

Raising injured part above level of heart lessens bleeding. If there is broken bone in limb, do not raise it until it has been properly splinted.

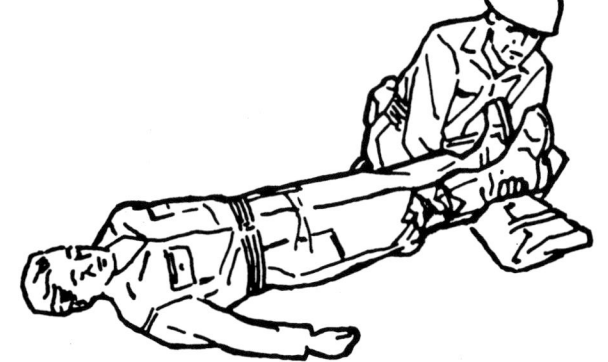

Digital Pressure (B)

(Pressure with fingers, thumbs, or hands)

If blood is spurting from wound (artery), press at the point or site where main artery supplying the wounded area lies near skin surface or over bone as shown below. This pressure shuts off or slows down the flow of blood from the heart to the wound until a pressure dressing can be unwrapped and applied. You will know you have located the artery when you feel a pulse.

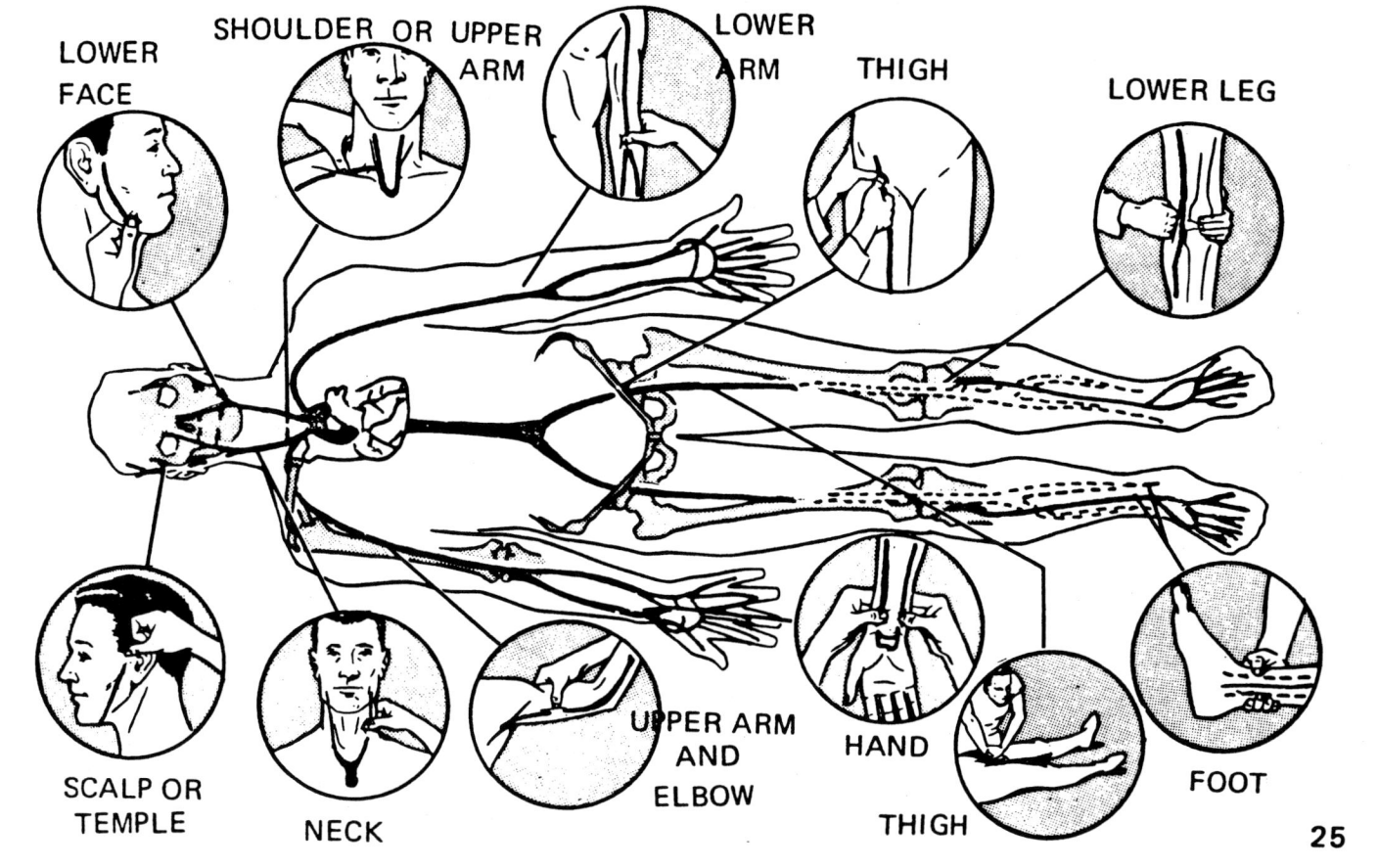

LOWER FACE

SHOULDER OR UPPER ARM

LOWER ARM

THIGH

LOWER LEG

SCALP OR TEMPLE

NECK

UPPER ARM AND ELBOW

HAND

THIGH

FOOT

25

Tourniquet (B)

Use tourniquet as last resort. Apply it between the wound and where the limb is attached to the body. Place it 2 to 4 inches above the injury, not over wound or fracture.
Never loosen or remove a tourniquet once you have applied it. If possible, mark a T on soldier's forehead and time you applied tourniquet. Get him to medical treatment facility as soon as possible.

(a)

Make a loop around the limb with any flexible material; tie with square knot.

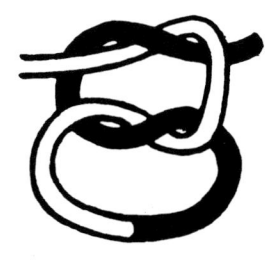

SQUARE KNOT

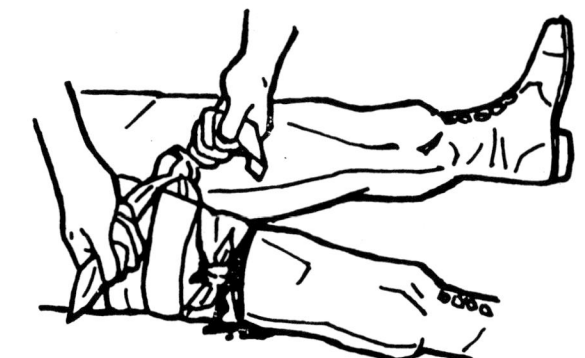

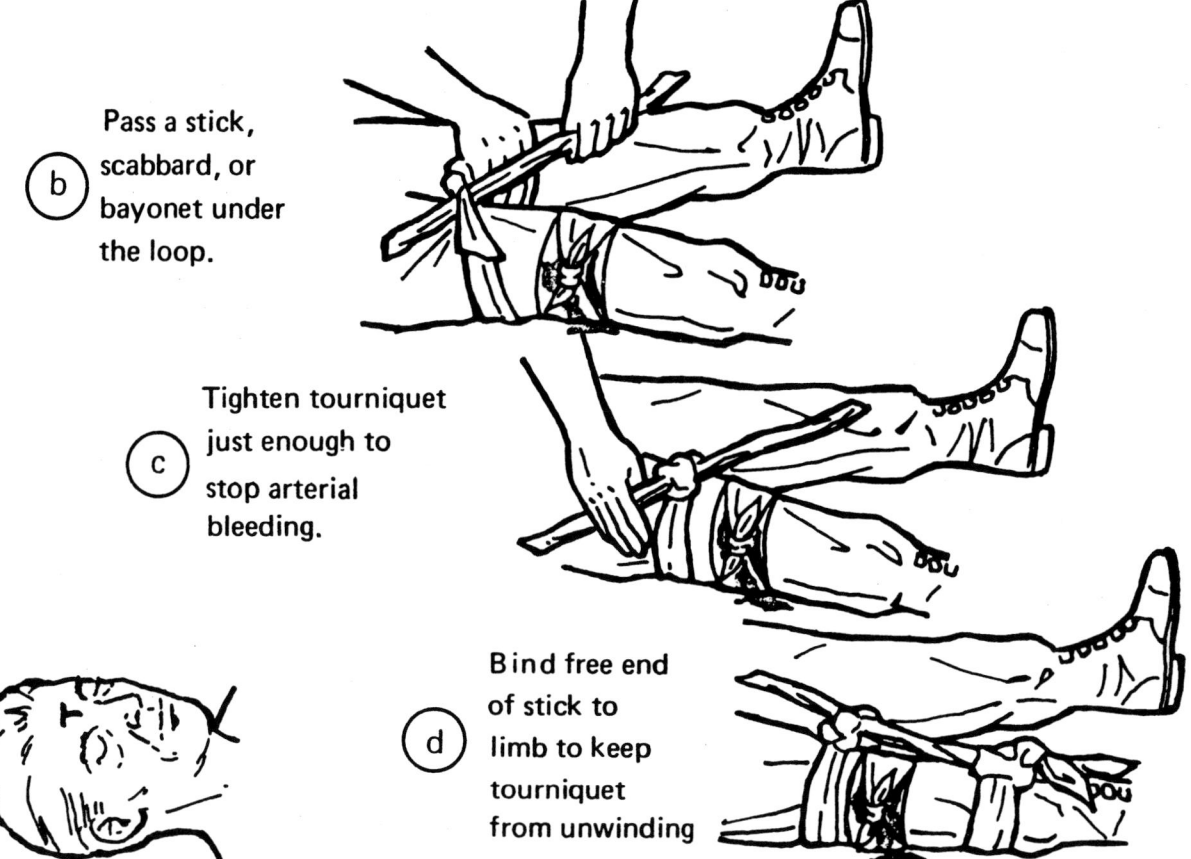

b Pass a stick, scabbard, or bayonet under the loop.

c Tighten tourniquet just enough to stop arterial bleeding.

d Bind free end of stick to limb to keep tourniquet from unwinding

27

PREVENT SHOCK (C)

Shock may result from any injury but is more likely to develop in severe injuries.

Warning signs:	May be:	Signs as shock get worse:
Restlessness	Excited or appear	Small fast breaths or gasps
Thirst	calm and tired	Staring vacantly into space
Paleness of skin	Sweating when skin	Blotchy or bluish skin,
Rapid heartbeat	feels cool and clammy	especially around mouth

1. **Maintain adequate respiration and heartbeat.**

   This may entail only clearing soldier's upper airway, positioning him to insure drainage of any fluid blocking airway, and observing him to insure airway remains clear. However, you may need to give him artificial respiration and closed-chest heart massage (pages 12-19.)

2. **Stop bleeding (pages 20-27).**

3. **Loosen tight clothing.**

   Loosen clothing at neck, waist, and other places where it tends to bind. Loosen, but do not remove shoes.

4. Reassure soldier.

Take charge. Show by your calm self-confidence and gentle yet firm actions that you know what you are doing and that you expect him to feel better because you are helping him. If he asks questions about the seriousness of his injury, explain that a physician will have to examine him to determine the extent of injury. Ill-timed or incorrect information can increase a person's anxiety.

5. Splint fractures (pages 44-48).

6. Position soldier.
(Splint any fracture first)
If conscious -- On back with feet raised 6" to 8".
If unconscious -- On side or abdomen with head turned to side.
Vary position for:
Head injury -- Head also raised higher than body.
Face and neck wound -- Sit, lean forward with head down or in unconscious position.
Sucking wound of chest -- Sit or lie on injured side.
Abdominal wound -- On back with head turned to side.

CONSCIOUS

UNCONSCIOUS

7. Keep soldier comfortably warm.
Place suitable material (poncho, blanket, etc.) under him as well as over him if weather makes necessary. If weather permits, remove any wet clothing except boots.

29

Protecting the wound as soon as possible from further contamination decreases possibilities for infection and increases casualty's chances for recovery.

Dressing . . . . A sterile pad or compress used to cover wound. It is usually made of gauze or cotton wrapped in gauze.

Bandage . . . . A strip or piece of gauze or muslin used over dressing to hold it in place, to close off dressing's edges from dirt and germs, and to create pressure on wound for control of bleeding. It is also used to support injured part or to hold splint to fractured part.

Field First Aid Dressing with attached bandages (D)

WRAPPED DRESSING (WITH ATTACHED BANDAGES) IN PLASTIC ENVELOPE

a After you cut and lift clothing from wound, remove wrapped dressing (with attached bandages) from plastic envelope; then twist to break paper wrapper.

b Grasp folded bandages with hands, being careful not to touch side of dressing which goes next to wound.

d Wrap bandages around the part and tie ends securely with square knot.

c Place dressing on wound without allowing it to touch anything else.

NOTE: The bandages attached to field first aid dressing are split 4-6 inches from the loose ends. They may be split farther to make four tails long enough for securing bandages around the head.

To make triangular bandages, cut a square of pliable material somewhat larger than 3 by 3 feet, fold it diagonally, and cut along fold. This makes two triangular bandages.

To make cravat bandages, fold each triangular bandage one, two, or three times, depending upon width desired.

Application of these bandages to some of the body parts is illustrated below.

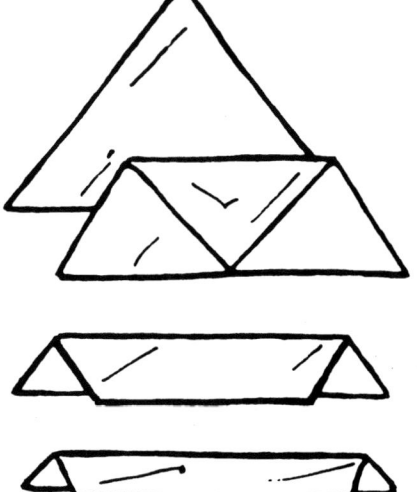

NOTE: To secure bandage in place, tie ends with square knot.

Triangular bandage applied to foot or hand (D)

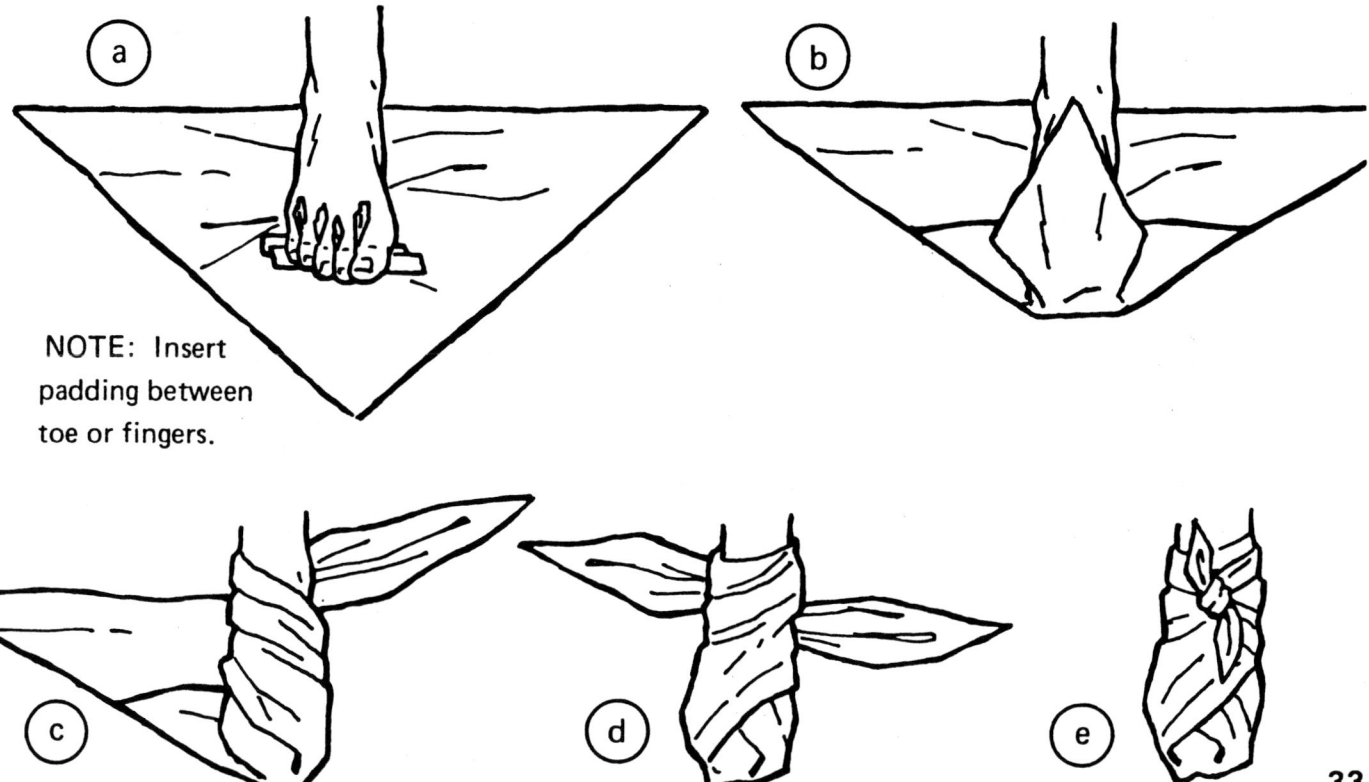

a

b

NOTE: Insert padding between toe or fingers.

c

d

e

33

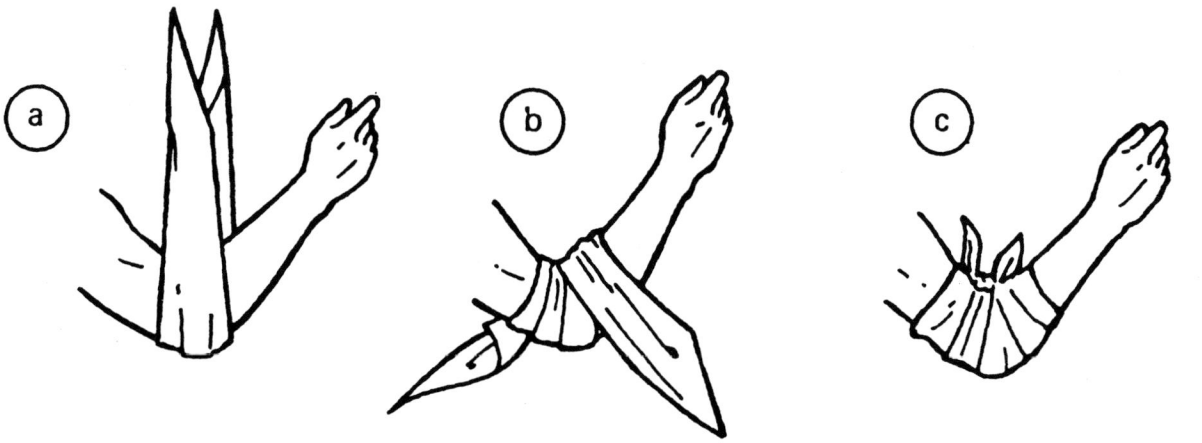

Cravat bandage applied to jaw (D)

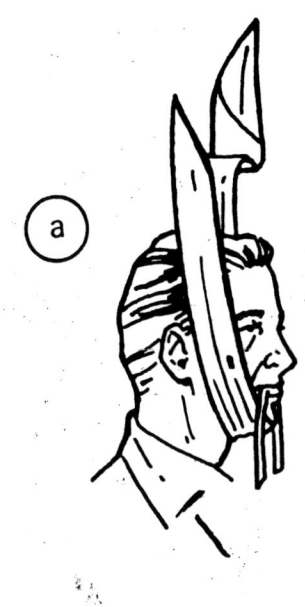

a

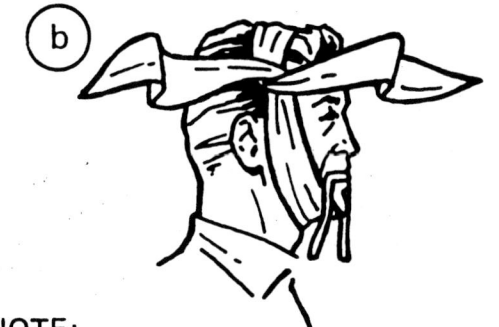

b

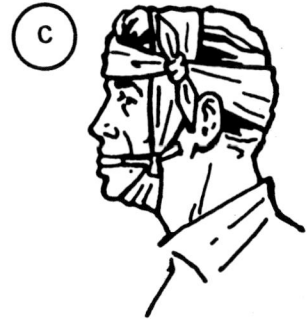

c

NOTE:

Before bandage jaw:
  Take any removable dentures from soldier's mouth and put them in his pocket.
Place wad of material (with streamers attached) between his teeth or gums.

After bandage jaw:
  Tie streamers to bandage.

Cravat bandage applied to ear or eye area (D)

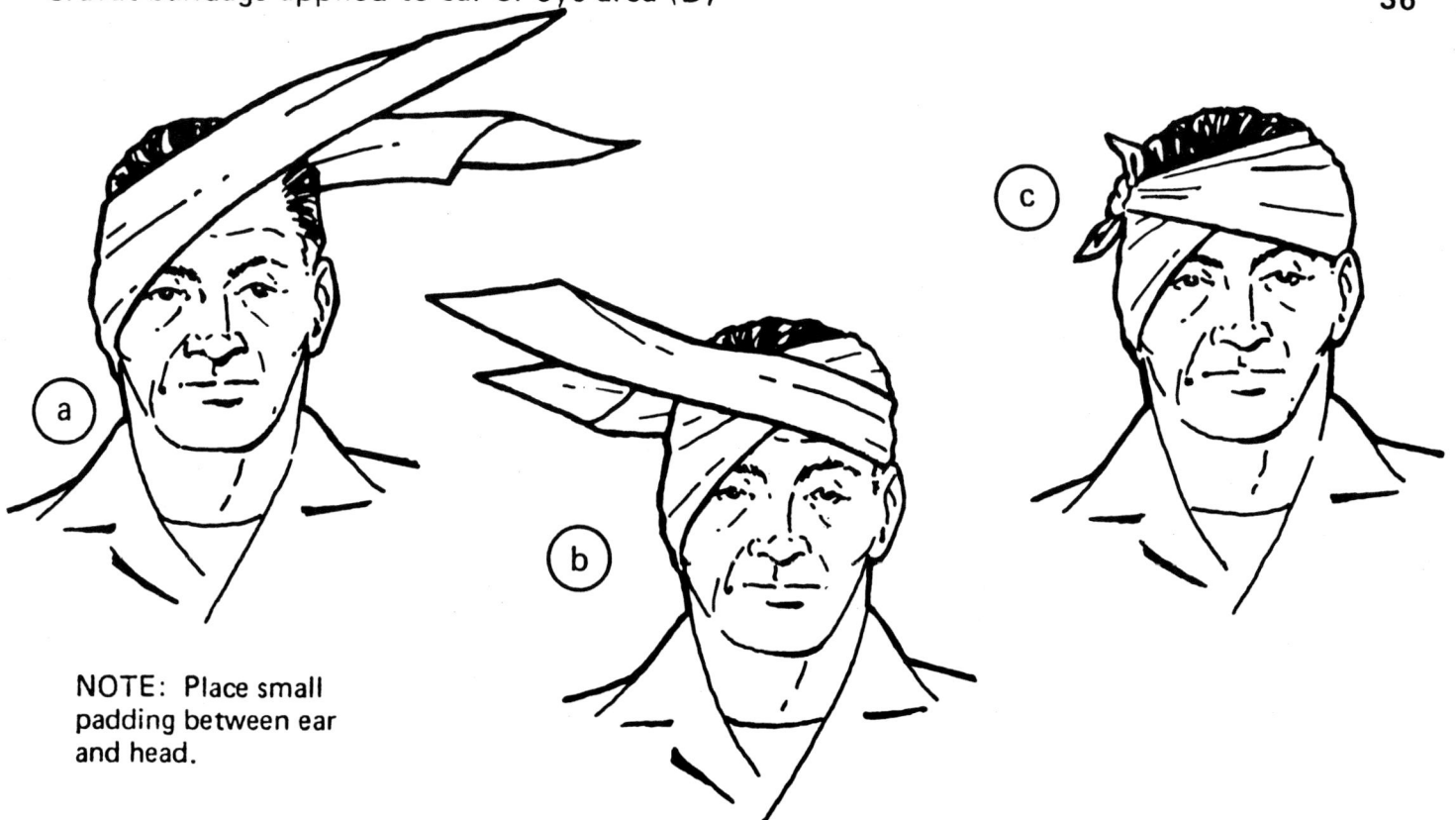

NOTE: Place small padding between ear and head.

PART 2

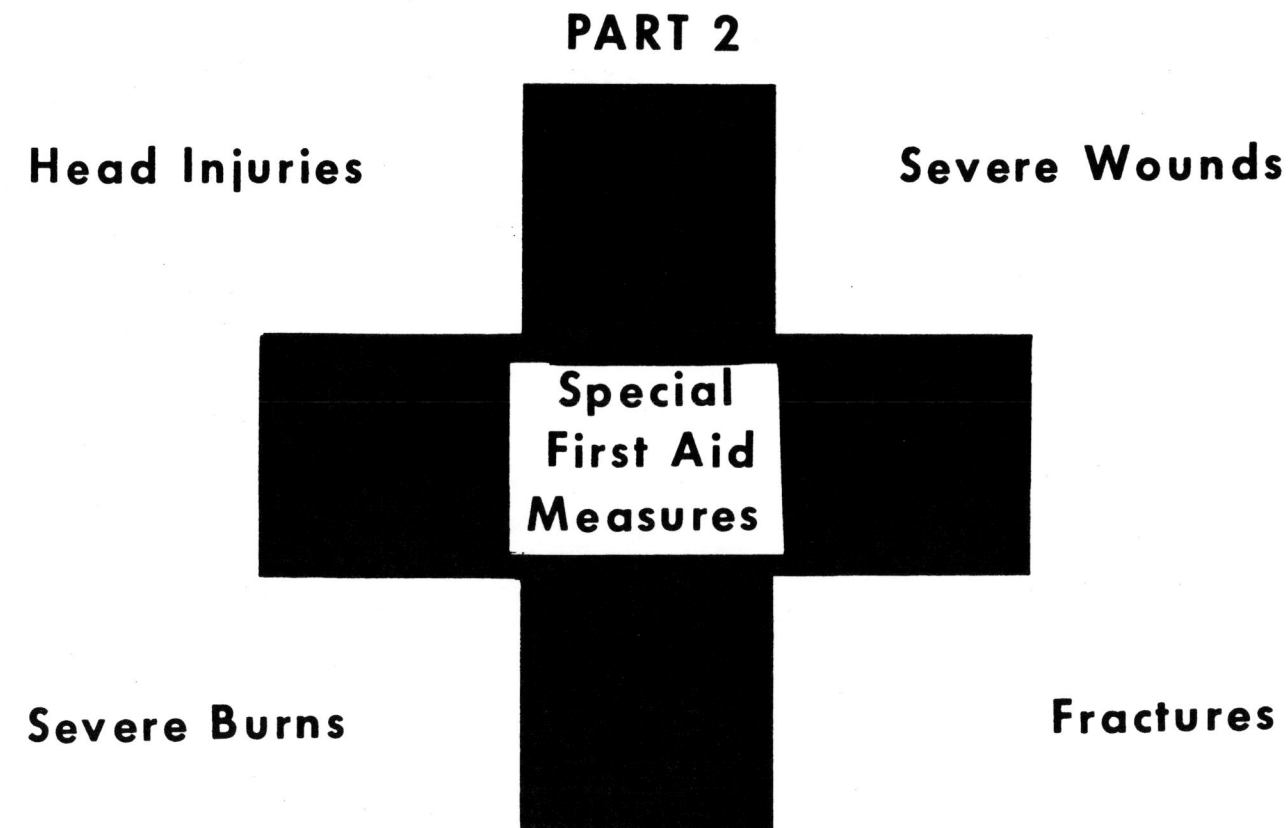

Head Injuries

Severe Wounds

Special First Aid Measures

Severe Burns

Fractures

Serious skull fractures and brain injuries usually occur together.

Signs:
Scalp wound.
If no scalp wound, check for other signs:
Is or has recently been unconscious.
Has blood or other fluid escaping from nose or ears.
Has slow pulse.
Has headache.
Is nauseated or is vomiting.
Has had convulsion.
Is breathing very slowly.

First Aid:
1. Leave any protruding brain tissue as it is and place a sterile dressing over this tissue. Do not remove or disturb any foreign matter which may be in the wound.
2. Secure dressing in place with bandages, using technique illustrated below.
3. Position soldier so that his head is higher than his body.

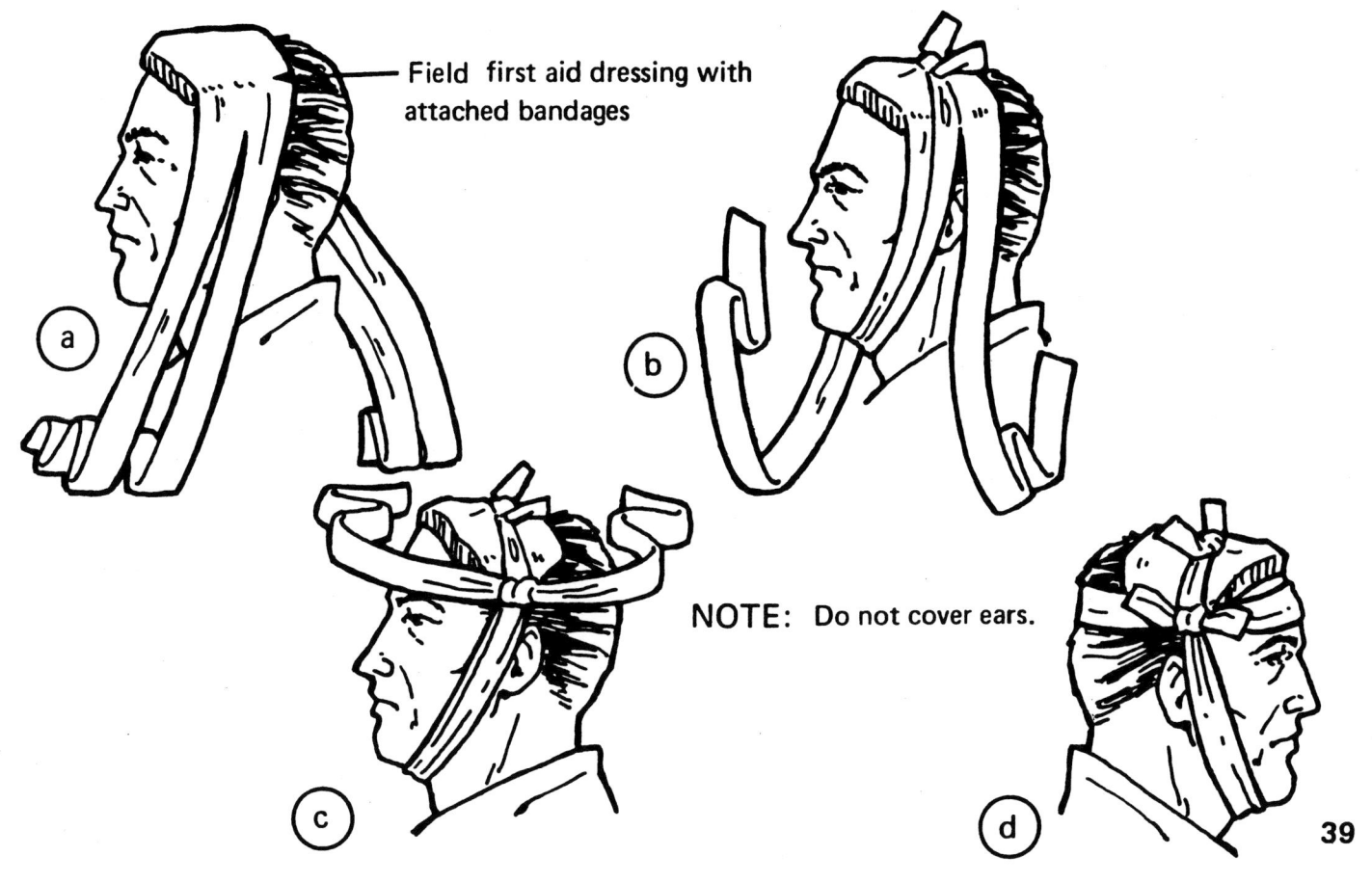

a — Field first aid dressing with attached bandages

b

c

NOTE: Do not cover ears.

d

Because of many blood vessels in area, bleeding is usually profuse and hard to control.

First Aid:

1. Stop bleeding causing obstruction of upper airway first.

2. Clear airway with your fingers, removing blood, mucus, any pieces of broken teeth or bone, bits of flesh, as well as dentures.

3. If casualty is conscious and wants to sit, have him lean forward with head down to permit drainage from mouth. Otherwise, place him on abdomen with head turned to side to permit drainage from mouth.

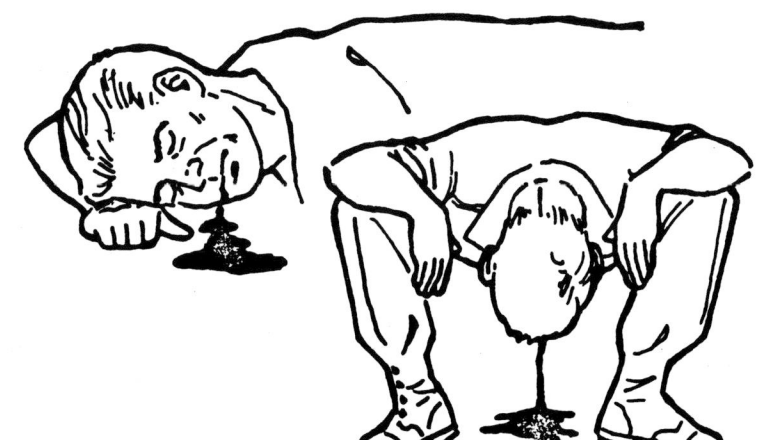

4. Evacuate as soon as possible.

CHEST WOUNDS

Wound which results in air being sucked into chest cavity causes lung on injured side to collapse.

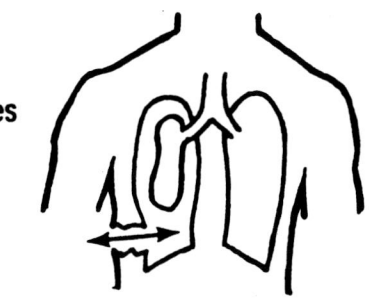

First Aid:

1. Have casualty forcibly breathe out, it possible, and hold breath while you seal wound.

2. Seal wound airtight with plastic wrapper from dressing or foil-lined envelope from burn solution (in first aid case).

3. Place field first aid dressing over plastic or foil.

4. Have casualty or another person press with open hand on dressing while you secure attached bandages around body.

5. Cover dressing completely with bandaging material (folded poncho or strip torn from clothing, shelter half, blanket) and wrap it around body to create more pressure, thus making wound airtight. Secure bandages with casualty's belts.

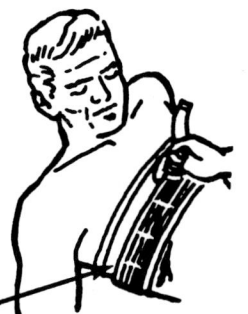

6. If casualty finds sitting more comfortable, allow him to do so. If he wants to lie down, encourage him to lie on injured side.

41

ABDOMINAL WOUNDS

An object may penetrate the abdominal wall and pierce internal organs or large blood vessels.

First Aid:

1. Leave protruding organs as they are and place sterile dressing over them.
2. Secure dressings in place with bandages, but do not apply them tightly, as internal bleeding cannot be controlled by pressure.
3. Do not allow casualty to take anything by mouth. Moisten lips to help lessen thirst.
4. Leave soldier on his back with his head turned to one side. Since he will likely vomit, watch him closely to prevent choking.

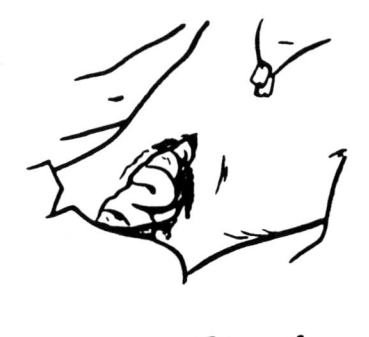

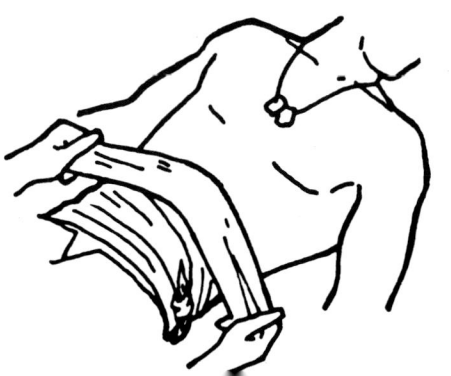

SEVERE BURNS

Primary objective is to prevent or lessen shock and infection.

First Aid:

1. If clothing is not stuck to the burn, cut clothing and lift it gently away without touching the burn.
2. Do NOT try to clean the burn in any way; DO NOT put any medication whatsoever on the burn.
3. Place sterile dressing over burned area and secure it in place with bandage. In mass casualty situation, use clean sheet in absence of sufficient dressings.
4. If soldier is conscious, is not vomiting, and has no abdominal or neck wound, give him the sodium chloride--sodium bicarbonate mixture from his first aid case. Dissolve one envelope of this mixture in one canteenful of cool (not warm) water. Give solution slowly: canteenful over period of one hour. If mixture is not available, dissolve one-half teaspoonful of salt and one-fourth teaspoonful of baking soda in one quart of cool water.

FRACTURES

Closed fracture: Break in bone without break in overlying skin.
Open fractures: Break in bone as well as overlying skin.

Fractures must be splinted (immobilized) to prevent razor-sharp edges of bone from moving and cutting tissue, muscle, blood vessels, and nerves; to reduce pain and help control shock; and to prevent closed fractures from becoming open fractures.

First Aid:

1. "Splint them where they lie"— Splint (immobilize) fractured part <u>without</u> changing position of part and <u>before</u> moving injured person. If bone is in unnatural position, do not straighten it. If person must be moved to save his life, such as from enemy fire or a burning building, tie fractured part to uninjured part, grasp him under arm pits and pull him in straight line.
2. Apply splint so joint above fracture and joint below fracture are immobilized.
3. Use padding between injured part and splint.
4. Secure splint to part with bandages at several points above and below fracture (NOT across fracture); tie bandages against splint with square knot.
5. Use sling to support splinted arm bent at elbow and fractured elbow which is bent.

Fractured Arm, Elbow, or Wrist

Fractured Arm or Elbow When Elbow Is Not Bent

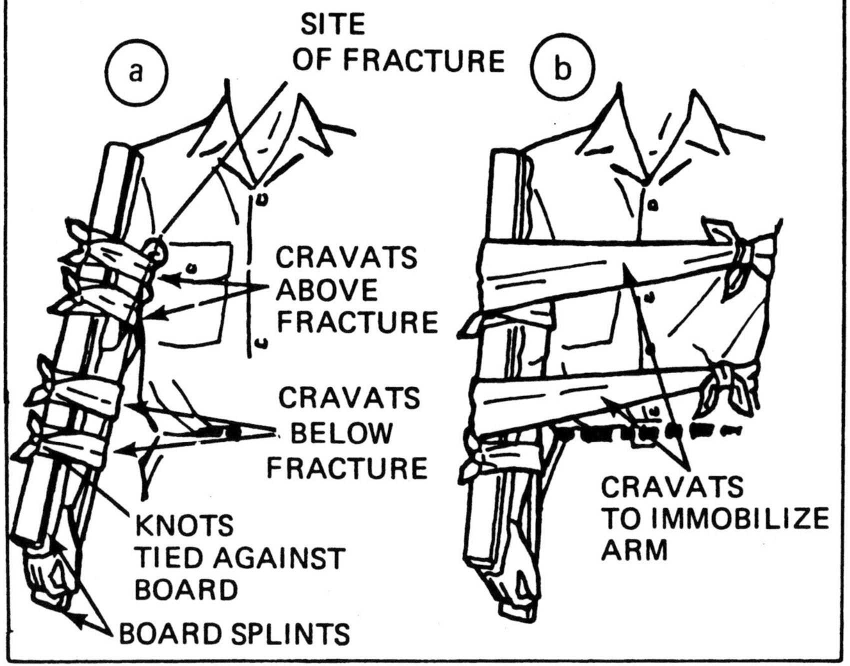

(a)

SITE OF FRACTURE

(b)

CRAVATS ABOVE FRACTURE

CRAVATS BELOW FRACTURE

KNOTS TIED AGAINST BOARD

BOARD SPLINTS

CRAVATS TO IMMOBILIZE ARM

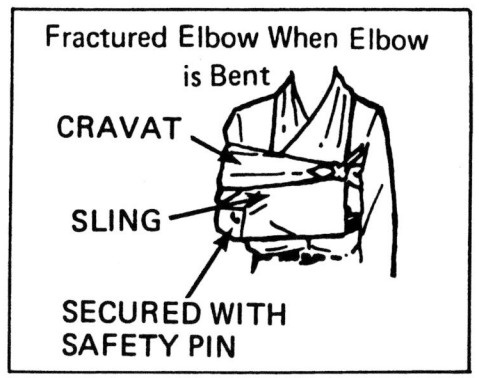

Fractured Elbow When Elbow is Bent

CRAVAT

SLING

SECURED WITH SAFETY PIN

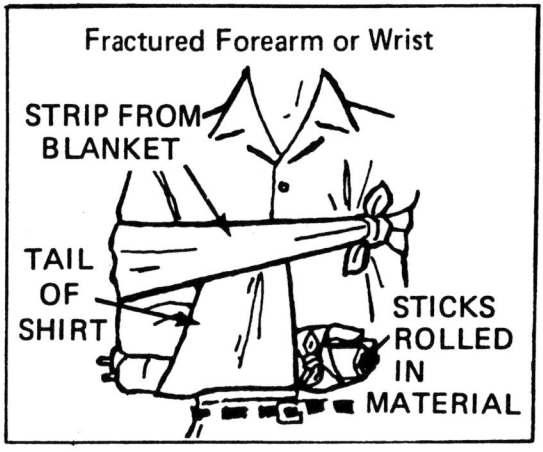

Fractured Forearm or Wrist

STRIP FROM BLANKET

TAIL OF SHIRT

STICKS ROLLED IN MATERIAL

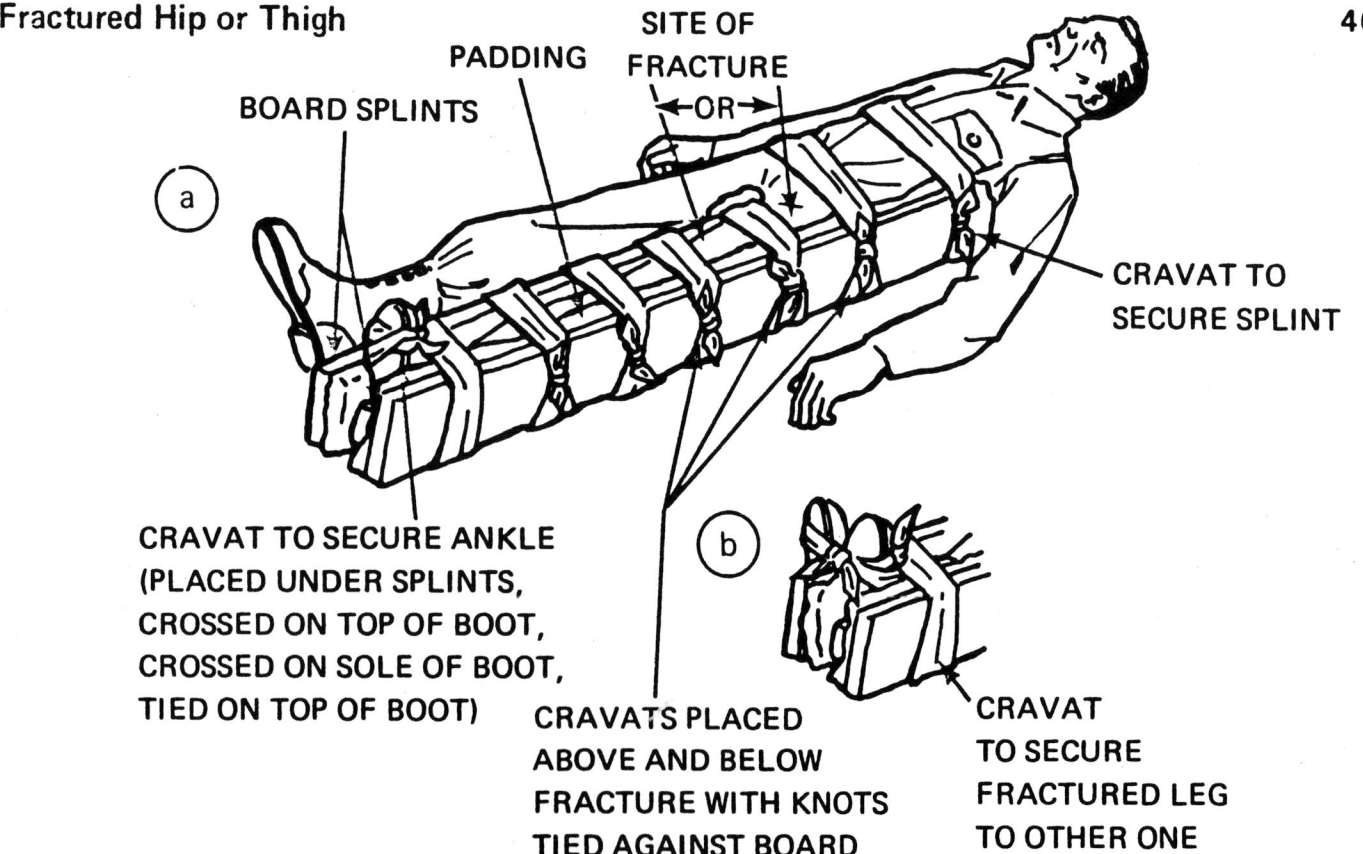

PADDING

SITE OF FRACTURE
←OR→

BOARD SPLINTS

CRAVAT TO SECURE SPLINT

a

CRAVAT TO SECURE ANKLE
(PLACED UNDER SPLINTS,
CROSSED ON TOP OF BOOT,
CROSSED ON SOLE OF BOOT,
TIED ON TOP OF BOOT)

b

CRAVATS PLACED
ABOVE AND BELOW
FRACTURE WITH KNOTS
TIED AGAINST BOARD

CRAVAT
TO SECURE
FRACTURED LEG
TO OTHER ONE

Fractured Lower Leg, Knee, or Ankle

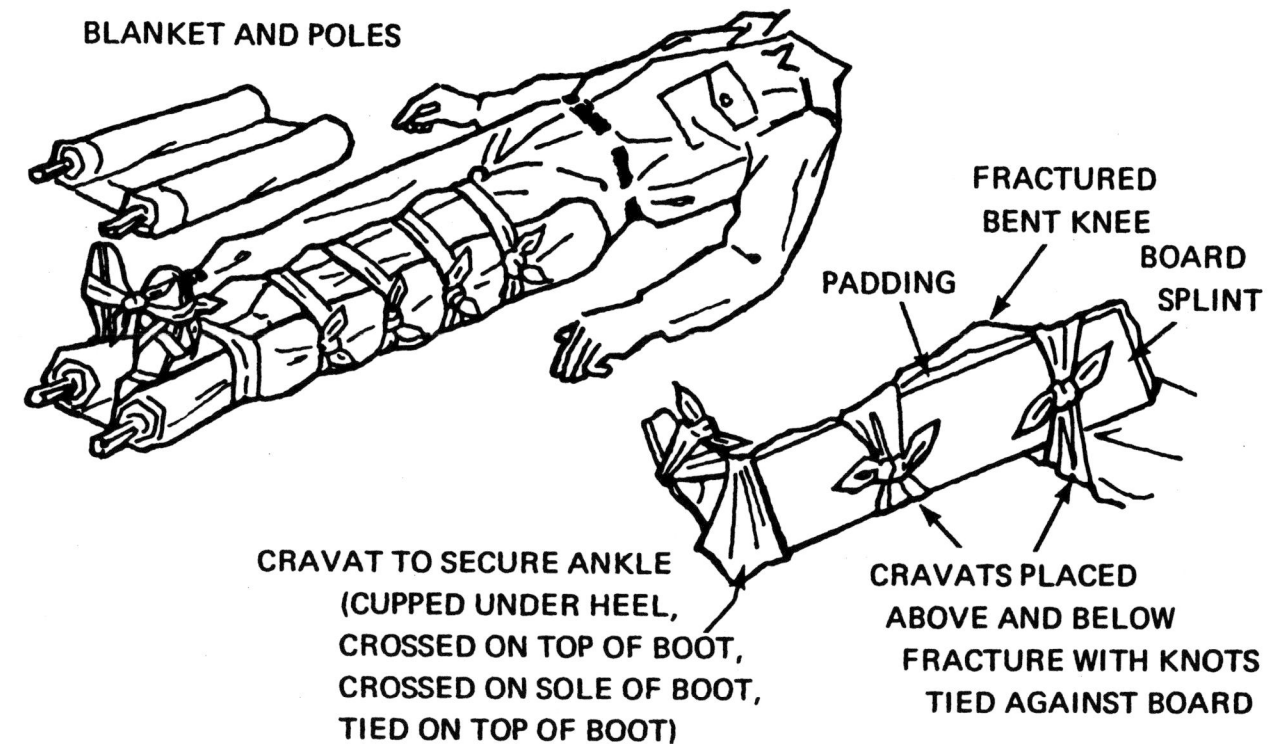

BLANKET AND POLES

FRACTURED BENT KNEE

PADDING

BOARD SPLINT

CRAVAT TO SECURE ANKLE
(CUPPED UNDER HEEL,
CROSSED ON TOP OF BOOT,
CROSSED ON SOLE OF BOOT,
TIED ON TOP OF BOOT)

CRAVATS PLACED
ABOVE AND BELOW
FRACTURE WITH KNOTS
TIED AGAINST BOARD

47

Fractured Back or Neck

If back, blanket under arch

If neck, small roll under neck

Neck: Steady head and neck, gently slide casualty onto board, slip roll under neck, and immobilize head.

Back: Tie wrists together loosely, place blanket on litter at arch site, gently lift casualty onto litter without bending his back.

PART 3

First Aid for Common Emergencies

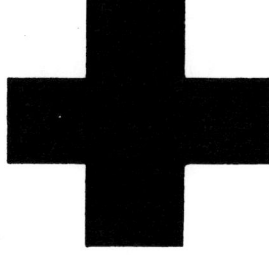

ABDOMINAL PAIN	SIGNS/SYMPTOMS	FIRST AID +	50
Appendicitis 	Pain in lower right or upper part of abdomen. May be nauseated or may vomit. Fever seldom present at first.	1. Withhold food and water. 2. DO NOT take laxative. 3. DO NOT heat abdomen. Ice bag over appendix area may relieve discomfort. 4. Get to medical treatment facility immediately.	
Hernia (Rupture) 	Bulge part way up groin from crotch. Bulge may appear in scar of abdominal operation, at navel, or just below groin at crotch. Some pain during first weeks, but less discomfort later.	1. Refrain from lifting vigorous activity. 2. DO NOT press on bulge. 3. If bulge does not subside when lying down, get to a medical treatment facility immediately. 4. If bulge disappears when lying down, continue to refrain from lifting and vigorous activity and get to medical treatment facility as soon as possible.	

CARBON MONOXIDE (CO) POISONING

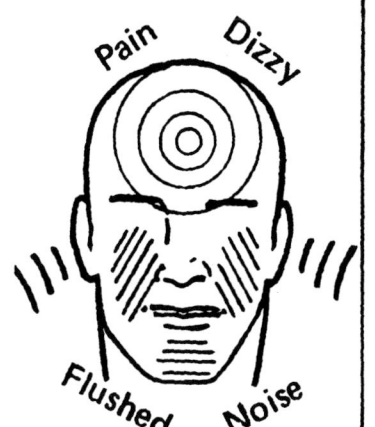

Pain · Dizzy · Flushed · Noise

SIGNS/SYMPTOMS	FIRST AID +
Dizziness, headache, noises in ears, throbbing in temples quickly followed by feelings of sleepiness and weakness. Vomiting and convulsions may occur, followed by unconsciousness and death. Skin and lips are often bright red.	1. Move him into fresh air immediately. 2. Give him artificial respiration. (It is SAFE to give mouth-to-mouth artificial respiration to a CO victim.) 3. Keep him quiet and transport him to medical treatment facility.

CHOKING
(Trachea obstructed by food)

SIGNS/SYMPTOMS	FIRST AID +

SIGNS/SYMPTOMS

Cannot breathe

Turns cyanotic (blue)

Collapses

(Has 4 minutes to live unless you relieve the obstruction.)

FIRST AID +

A. If victim is standing or sitting, apply the Heimlich hug as follows:
1. Stand behind him and wrap your arms around his waist.
2. Make fist with one hand and place it against his abdomen slightly above navel and below rib cage; then grasp wrist of this hand with other hand.
3. Press fist forcefully into his abdomen with quick upward thrust, causing sharp exhalation of air to blow food out airway.
4. Repeat several times, if necessary.

B. If victim is lying on his back, apply the Heimlich maneuver as follows:
1. Facing him, kneel astride his hips.
2. With one hand on top of other one, place heel of bottom hand on his abdomen slightly above navel and below rib cage.
3. Press forcefully with heel of hand into abdomen with quick upward thrust.
4. Repeat several times, if necessary.

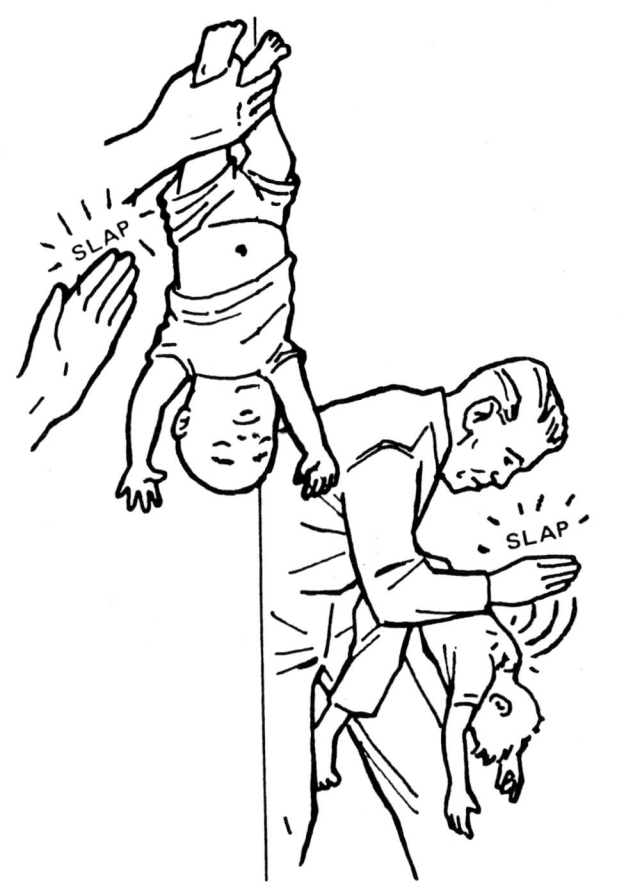

Baby:

1. Hold upside down with head hanging straight down.
2. Open mouth and pull tongue forward.
3. Should object not come out, reach in back of throat with index finger.
4. If still does not dislodge, slap baby sharply between shoulder blades.
5. If object does not come out, begin artificial respiration immediately.

Child:

1. Hold over arm or leg with head down.
2. Slap hard several times between shoulder blades.
3. Clear throat with index finger.
4. If difficulty in breathing continues, start artificial respiration.

53

DROWNING

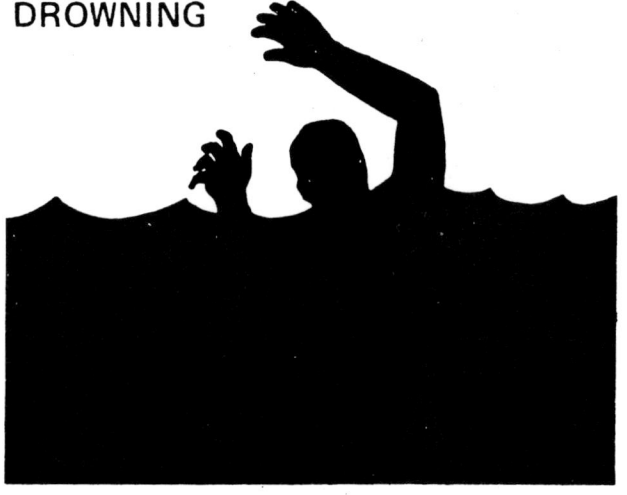

DO NOT enter water to attempt rescue
if you are not trained to do so.
Instead, toss end of rope or life preserver
or get end of long pole or branch to
struggling victim.

1. If you enter water to rescue victim, get his head above water.

2. As soon as his head is clear of water, start artificial respiration. Speed is essential.

3. If other rescuers can help carry him ashore, do not interrupt artificial respiration.

4. Once victim is ashore, do not waste valuable seconds turning him over to drain water from his lungs; continue artificial respiration.

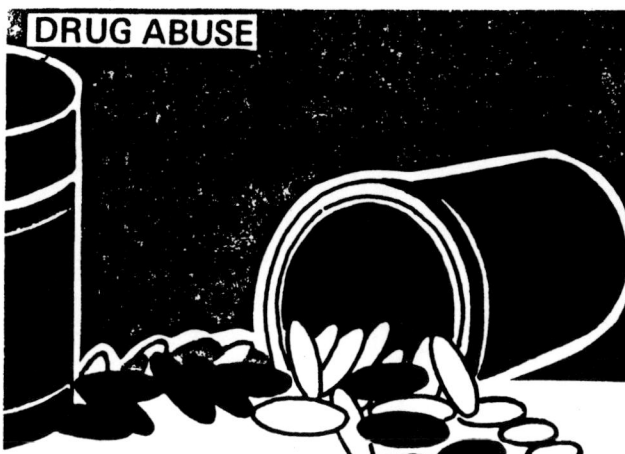

DRUG ABUSE

Symptoms of overdose:

"Uppers" -- Anxiety, overactivity, and fear. Usually eyes are dilated, and pulse and respiration are fast. May be trembling.

"Downers" -- Sluggish to unconscious condition, even stoppage of heartbeat and breathing. If drug is narcotic, pupils may be pinpoints. If awake, may have appearance of alcoholic intoxication without odor. Speech is usually slurred.

First aid for overdose of drugs depends upon whether they were "uppers" (stimulants) or "downers" (sedatives).
Regardless, get person to medical treatment facility immediately.

1. Try to calm person down; reassure him by your calm self-confidence and your gentle, yet firm actions.
2. DO NOT give coffee, tea, soda pop, or any liquid with caffein, as it will only stimulate him further.

1. Try to get him awake.
2. If not fully awake, keep his airway open.
3. Even though you are able to wake him, get him to medical treatment facility, as he could have serious relapse.

55

ELECTRIC SHOCK from electric current or lightening

Turn off switch if person is still in contact with electric current but do not waste time looking for switch. Instead, remove person from wire, using dry wooden pole, dry clothing, dry rope, or other material which will not conduct electricity.

DO NOT touch wire or person with your bare hands, as you will also get a shock.

1. Give person artificial respiration immediately after freeing him from electric wire, as electric shock causes breathing to stop.

2. Check pulse, as electric shock may also cause heart to stop. If you do not feel pulse immediately, give closed-chest heart massage with artificial respiration.

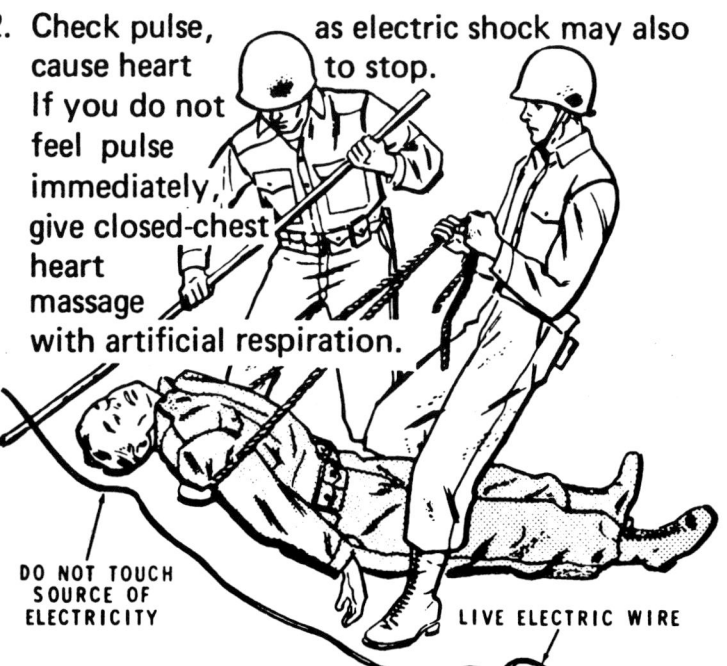

DO NOT TOUCH SOURCE OF ELECTRICITY

LIVE ELECTRIC WIRE

FOREIGN BODY IN EYE

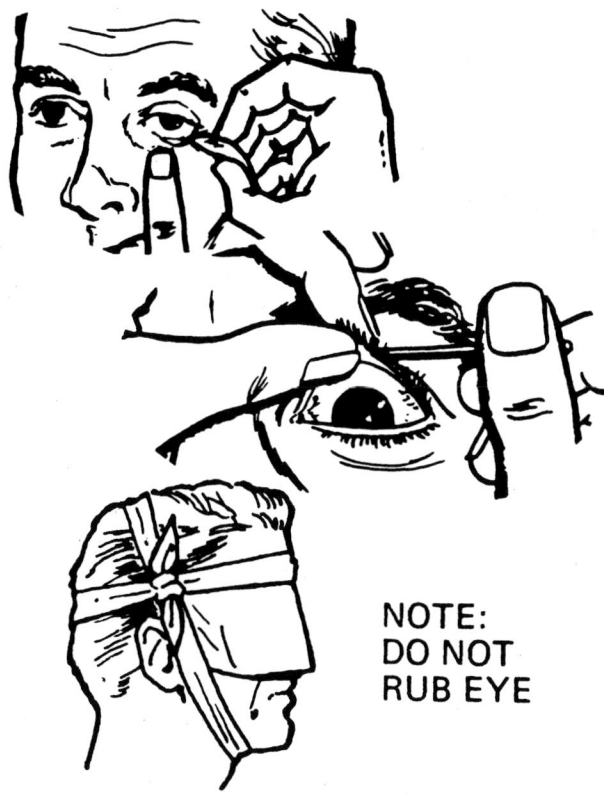

NOTE:
DO NOT
RUB EYE

1. If particle is beneath lower lid, gently remove it with moist clean corner of handkerchief.

2. If particle is beneath upper lid, grasp eyelashes and pull lid away from eyeball. Hold until tears start flowing freely and flush out the particle. If particle does not flush out, grasp eyelashes with thumb and finger; place match or twig over lid and pull lid over it; examine inside of lid while person looks down. Gently remove particle with clean corner of handkerchief.

3. If foreign particle is glass or metal or cannot be removed as indicated above, bandage both eyes and get him to medical treatment facility. Both eyes are bandaged to prevent movement of injured eye, since eyes have synchronized movements.

57

Black Widow Spider
or
Brown Recluse Spider
Bite

1. Keep victim quiet.
2. Place ice or freeze-pack, if available, around region of body where bite occurred to keep venom from spreading.
3. Transport him to medical treatment facility without delay.

Scorpion Sting
or
Tarantula Bite

1. For ordinary scorpion sting or tarantula bite, apply ice or freeze-pack, if available. Baking soda applied as paste to site may relieve pain.
2. If site of sting or bite is on face, neck, or genital organs or if sting is by scorpion of dangerous types found in South America, keep victim as quiet as possible and transport him to medical treatment facility without delay.

Snake Bite

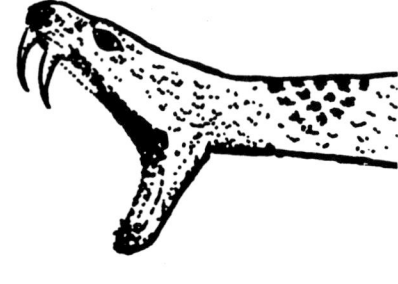

1. Reassure victim and keep him quiet.
2. Place ice or freeze-pack, if available, around region of body where bite occurred.
3. Immobilize affected part in position below level of heart.
4. If bite is on arm or leg, place lightly constricting band (bootlace, strip of cloth, etc.) between bite site and heart at point 2-4 inches above bite site. Apply band tightly enough to stop blood flow near skin but **NOT** tightly enough to stop arterial flow or the pulse.
5. Transport victim to medical treatment facility at once. Kill snake (if possible, without damaging its head) and evacuate with victim.

SUN OR HEAT INJURIES	SIGNS/SYMPTOMS	FIRST AID +
Heat Cramps	Muscle cramps of abdomen, legs, or arms.	1. Move person to shade and loosen clothing. 2. Give him large amounts of cool salt water slowly. Prepare salt water by dissolving 2 salt tablets or ¼ teaspoonful of table salt in canteen of cool water.
Heat Exhaustion	Headache, excessive sweating, weakness, dizziness, nausea, muscle cramps. Pale, cool, moist, clammy skin.	1. Lay person in cool shaded area and loosen his clothing. 2. If he is conscious, have him drink 3 to 5 canteenfuls of cool salt water during period of 12 hours. Prepare salt water as described for "heat cramps."
Heatstroke (Sunstroke) 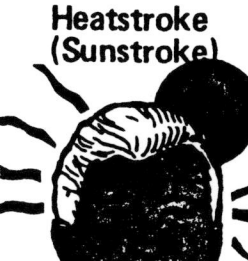	Stoppage of sweating (hot, dry skin). Collapse and unconsciousness may come suddenly or may be preceded by headache, dizziness, fast pulse, nausea, vomiting, and mental confusion.	1. Promptly immerse person in coldest water available. Add ice, if available, to water. If cannot immerse him, get him into shade, remove his clothing, keep his entire body wet by pouring water over him, and fan his wet body continuously. 2. Transport him to nearest medical facility at once, cooling his body on way. 3. If he becomes conscious, give him cool salt water prepared as described for "heat cramps."

1. Apply Lifesaving Measures A,B,C,D as appropriate.

2. If person remain unconscious, place him on his abdomen or side with head turned to one side to prevent his choking on vomitus, blood, or other fluid. If he has abdominal wound, place him on back with head turned to one side. Get person to medical treatment facility immediately.

3. DO NOT give him fluids by mouth while he is unconscious.

4. If he has merely fainted, he will regain consciousness within a few minutes. If ammonia inhalant capsule is available, break it and place it under his nose several times for a few seconds. If he is sitting, gently lay him down, loosen his clothing, apply cool wet cloth to his face, and let him lie quietly. Anytime a person in sitting position is about to faint, lower his head between his knees and hold him to prevent his falling.

WET OR COLD INJURIES	SIGNS/SYMPTOMS	FIRST AID +
Frostbite	Skin is white, stiff, and numb.	1. Cover frostbitten part of face with warm hands until pain returns. 2. Place frostbitten bare hands next to skin in opposite armpits. 3. If feet are frostbitten, seek sheltered area and place bare feet under clothing and against abdomen of another person. 4. If deep frostbite is suspected, protect part from additional injury and get to medical treatment facility by fastest means possible. DO NOT attempt to thaw deep frostbite. There is less danger of walking on feet while frozen than after thawed.
Immersion Foot	Soles of feet are wrinkled. Standing or walking is extremely painful.	1. Dry feet thoroughly and get to medical treatment facility by fastest means possible. 2. Avoid walking if possible.
Trench Foot	Numbness. May be tingling or aching sensation, cramping pain, and swelling.	Same as for "Immersion Foot" above.
Snow Blindness	Scratchy feeling in eyes.	1. Cover eyes with dark cloth. 2. Transport him to medical treatment facility at once.

Blisters

DO NOT open blisters unnecessarily, as they are sterile until opened. If you must open blister, be cautious:

1. Wash part thoroughly with soap and water; then apply antiseptic to skin.
2. Sterilize a needle in the open flame of a match, etc.
3. Using sterile needle, puncture blister at its edge.
4. Using sterile gauze pad, apply pressure along margin of blister, thus removing fluid.
5. Place a sterile dressing over the area.

DO NOT attempt self help for blisters in the center palm of hand.

Boils

1. DO NOT squeeze a boil, as this may drive bacteria into the blood stream and cause internal abscesses or bone infection. This is especially unwise if boil is around nostrils, upper lip, or area of the eyes, as here the blood stream leads to brain area.
2. Relieve discomfort from small boils by applying warm compresses wet in Epsom salt solution (one teaspoon salt to pint of warm water) at 15-minute intervals. DO NOT apply these compresses to facial boils unless under medical direction.
3. If boil breaks, wipe pus away with sterile pad wet with rubbing alcohol. Work from healthy skin toward boil and pus.
4. Apply sterile dressing over boil.

NOTES

NOTES